C000241272

KETO MEAL PLAN #2021

An Essential Guide to
Follow Step by Step with
Tasty & Easy Recipes
Homemade by Anyone

by **TAMARA GREEN**

Congratulation on purchase this book and thank You for doing so.

Please enjoy!

© Copyright 2021 by **TAMARA GREEN**

All Rights Reserved

Table of Contents

Chapter 1

Delicious Breakfast Dishes

From eggs to sweet goodies, you are sure to find a perfect breakfast dish here!

Eggs Delight

Almost Mc Griddle Casserole

Serving Yields: 8

Macros: 3 g Net Carbs | 448 Calories | 26 g Protein | 36 g Total Fats

Fixings Needed:

- Breakfast sausage - 1 lb.
- Flaxseed meal - .25 cup
- Almond flour - 1 cup
- Large eggs - 10
- Maple syrup - 6 tbsp.
- Cheese - 4 oz.
- Butter - 4 tbsp.
- Onion - .5 tsp.
- Garlic powder - .5 tsp.
- Sage - .25 tsp.
- Also Needed: 9 x 9-inch casserole dish

How to Prepare:

- Heat up the oven temperature to 350ºF.
- Use the medium heat setting on the stovetop to prepare the sausage in a skillet. Add all of the dry ingredients (the cheese also) and stir in the wet ones. Add 4 tablespoons of the syrup. Stir and blend well.
- After the sausage is browned, combine all of the fixings along with the grease.
- Prepare the casserole dish with a sheet of parchment paper. Empty the mix into the casserole dish and drizzle the rest of the syrup on the top.
- Bake for 45-55 minutes.
- Transfer to the countertop and let it become room temperature. The casserole should be easy to remove by using the edge of the parchment paper.

Meal Prep Tips:

1. After the casserole has cooled, just slice it into 8 portions.
2. You can enjoy for a couple of days.
3. You can also freeze the rest for later.

Avocado & Eggs

Serving Yields: 2

Macros: 9 g Net Carbs | 275 Calories | 8 g Protein | 23 g Total Fats

Fixings Needed:

- Eggs - 2
- Avocado - 1 ripened
- Optional: Hot sauce
- Salt & Freshly cracked black pepper - to your liking

How to Prepare:

1. Warm up the oven until it reaches 425ºF.
2. Slice the avocado in half and discard the pit. Use a metal scoop to remove about 1-2 tablespoons of the fleshy insides. Arrange the halves in a small baking pan. Crack an egg into both halves and season with some pepper and salt.
3. Bake 15-20 minutes.

Meal Prep Tips:

1. Let the fixings cool and store for a day or so in the refrigerator to enjoy the next morning or for a snack.
2. If you want to spice it up a little, sprinkle in a portion of keto-friendly hot sauce on the second day.

Bacon Cheese & Egg Cups

Serving Yields: 6
Macros: 1 g Net Carbs | 101 Calories | 8 g
Protein | 7 g Total Fats

Fixings Needed:
- Large eggs - 6
- Bacon - 6 strips
- Cheese - .25 cup
- Fresh spinach - 1 handful
- Pepper & Salt - to taste

How to Prepare:
1. Warm up the oven to 400ºF.
2. Prepare the bacon using medium heat on the stovetop. Place on towels to drain.
3. Grease 6 muffin tins with a spritz of oil.
4. Line each tin with a slice of bacon, pressing tightly to make a secure well for the eggs.
5. Drain and dry the spinach with a paper towel. Whisk the eggs and combine with the spinach.
6. Add the mixture to the prepared tins and sprinkle with cheese. Sprinkle with salt and pepper until it's like you like it.
7. Bake for 15 minutes. Remove when done and cool.

Meal Prep Tips:
1. Prepare the cups and store in airtight containers.
2. Reheat when ready to eat. It keeps in the fridge for 3-4 days.

Baked Greek Eggs

Servings: 6

Macros: 175 Calories | 5 g Net Carbs | 11 g Total Fats | 15 g Protein

Fixings Needed:
- Sun-dried tomatoes - .25 cup
- Feta cheese - .5 cup
- Oregano - .5 tsp.
- Chopped kale - 1 cup
- Eggs - 12

How to Prepare:
- Warm up the oven to reach 350ºF.
- Cover a baking tin with foil and a spritz of nonstick cooking spray.

- Whisk the eggs and combine with the rest of the fixings. Stir into the prepared pan. Bake for 25 minutes.
- Transfer to the countertop to completely cool. Slice.

Meal Prep Tips:
1. Store in the refrigerator for 4-5 days in an airtight container.
2. You can also place them into individual portions.

Spinach Quiche

Serving Yields: 6
Macros: -0- g Net Carbs | 299 Calories | 19.4 g Protein | 23 g Total Fats

Fixings Needed:
- Chopped onion - 1
- Olive oil - 1 tbsp.
- Frozen & thawed spinach - 1 pkg. 10 oz.
- Shredded Muenster cheese - 3 cups
- Organic eggs - whisked - 5
- To Taste: Black pepper and salt
- Also Needed: 9-inch pie plate

How to Prepare:
1. Warm up the oven to reach 350°F. Lightly grease the dish.
2. Use the medium heat setting to warm a skillet with the oil. Toss in the onion and sauté for 4-5 minutes. Raise the heat setting to medium-high.
3. Add the spinach and sauté for two to three minutes until the liquid is absorbed. Cool slightly
4. Combine the rest of the fixings in a large bowl and mix with the cooled spinach. Dump into the prepared dish and bake for 30 minutes.
5. Take the quiche out of the oven and cool for at least ten minutes.
6. Slice into six wedges.

Meal Prep Tips:
1. Add the cooled pieces into plastic baggies.
2. It will store in the fridge for two to four days.
3. To warm up, just prepare in the microwave for one minute on the high setting before serving.

Tomato & Cheese Frittata

Serving Yields: 2

Macros: 6 g Net Carbs | 435 Calories | 27 g Protein | 33 g Total Fats

Fixings Needed:
- Eggs - 6
- Soft cheese - 3.5 oz. - .66 cup
- White onion - .5 of 1 medium
- Halved cherry tomatoes - .66 cup
- Chopped herbs - ex. Chives or basil - 2 tbsp.
- Ghee or butter - 1 tbsp.

How to Prepare:
1. Set the oven broiler temperature to 400ºF.
2. Arrange the onions on a greased - hot iron skillet. Cook with either the ghee or butter until lightly browned.
3. In another dish, crack the eggs and flavor with the salt, pepper, or add some herbs of your choice. Whisk and add to the pan of onions, cooking until the edges begin to get crispy.
4. Top with the cheese (such as feta) and a few diced tomatoes. Put the pan in the broiler for five to seven minutes or until done.
5. Enjoy piping hot or let cool down.

6. Note: You can purge all of the leftover veggies into the recipe (if you wish).

Meal Prep Tips:
1. Divide into two equal portions. Place in separate containers until you're ready to enjoy a healthy breakfast.
2. Enjoy this readily prepared frittata that you can serve either hot or cold.
3. The deliciously prepared frittata will store in the fridge for up to five days. So, prep enough for several days.

<u>Other Delicious Choices</u>

Apple Banana Muffins

Serving Yields: 12
Macros: 8 g Net Carbs | 134 Calories | 11 g Protein | 4 g Total Fats

Fixings Needed:
- Baking powder - 1 tsp.
- Salt - .25 tsp.
- Baking soda - .5 tsp.
- Egg - 1
- Olive oil - 3 tbsp.
- Vanilla extract - 1 tsp.
- Unsweetened applesauce - .5 cup
- Ripe bananas - 1.5 cups
- Whole wheat flour - 1.33 cups

How to Prepare:
1. Heat up the oven to 375ºF. Heavily grease a muffin tin.
2. Whisk the egg and add the mashed bananas. Stir in everything but the flour.

3. Next, fold in the flour, being careful not to overmix. Pour into the muffin tin and bake for approximately 20-25 minutes.

Meal Prep Tips:
1. When the muffins are done, transfer them to the countertop and cool in the pan for about 5 minutes. At that time, arrange them on a cooling rack to thoroughly cool before proceeding.
2. Place the muffins in a storage container or freezer baggie.
3. Store in the fridge for about 5 days or freeze for later.

Blueberry Pancake Bites

Serving Yields: 24 bites
Macros: 7.5 g Net Carbs | 188 Calories | 6 g Protein | 13 g Total Fats

Fixings Needed:
- Baking powder - 1 tsp
- Water - .33 - .5 cup
- Melted ghee - .25 cup
- Coconut flour - .5 cup
- Cinnamon - .5 tsp.
- Salt - .5 tsp.

- Eggs - 4
- Vanilla extract - .5 tsp.
- Frozen blueberries - .5 cup
- Also Needed: Muffin tray

How to Prepare:
1. Warm up the oven to reach 325ºF. Use a spritz of coconut oil spray to grease 24 muffin cups.
2. Combine the eggs, sweetener, and vanilla; mixing until smooth. Fold in the flour, melted ghee, salt, baking powder, and cinnamon. Stir in .33 cup of water to finish the batter.
3. The mixture should be thick. Next, divide the batter into the prepared cups with several berries in each one.
4. Bake until set (20-25 min.). Cool.

Meal Prep Tips:
1. Store in an airtight container, preferably cool also.
2. It will be good for 8-10 days.
3. Freeze for 60-80 days.

Cheddar-Jalapeno Waffles

Serving Yields: 1
Macros: 6 g Net Carbs | 338 Calories | 16 g Protein | 28 g Total Fats

Fixings Needed:
- Large eggs - 3
- Jalapeno - 1 small
- Cream cheese - 3 oz.
- Coconut flour - 1 tbsp.
- Cheddar cheese - 1 oz.
- Baking powder - 1 tsp.
- Psyllium husk powder - 1 tsp.

How to Prepare:
1. Mix all of the ingredients using an immersion blender except for the jalapeno and cheese.
2. After you have a smooth texture, add the cheese and jalapeno. Blend and pour the batter into the waffle iron.
3. Cook for 5-6 minutes. Set aside when done.

Meal Prep Tips:

1. Let the waffles cool off for prep.
2. Put them into a plastic freezer bag. Store them in the freezer until you have the desire for a delicious waffle.
3. To reheat, preheat the oven temperature to 400ºF. When it's hot, place the waffles on a baking tin. Warm them up for 5 minutes. Serve and enjoy!
4. Tip: It isn't recommended to warm them in a regular toaster.

Note: These delicious waffles are complemented by psyllium husk which is a native of Pakistan, Bangladesh, and India. Its fiber content is right for your gut as a bulk-forming laxative which is useful in the keto diet since constipation can be one of the side effects.

French Style Crepes

Serving Yields: 2
Macros: 5 g Net Carbs | 319 Calories | 8 g Protein | 27.4 g Total Fats

Fixings Needed:
- Organic eggs - 2
- Melted coconut oil - divided – 2 tbsp.
- Sea salt - .125 tsp.

- Splenda - 1 tsp.
- Coconut flour - 2 tbsp.
- Heavy cream - .33 cup

How to Prepare:
1. Whisk the eggs, 1 tablespoon of oil, salt, and Splenda.
2. Slowly add the flour, whisking until well mixed. Stir in the cream.
3. Use the rest of the oil to grease a pan. Empty in 1/4 of the mixture and tilt the skillet to make a thin layer. Cook for two minutes, flip, and cook one more minute.
4. Proceed with the rest of the egg mixture to make the four crepes. Cool thoroughly.

Meal Prep Tips:
1. Wrap each one in plastic. Store in the fridge for up to two days.
2. Simply reheat in the microwave for 30 seconds when ready to use.

Pancakes & Nuts

Serving Yields: 2
Macros: 9 g Net Carbs | 625 Calories | 27 g Protein | 52 g Total Fats

Fixings Needed:
- Almond flour - 10 tbsp.
- Ground cinnamon - 1 tsp.
- Baking soda - .5 tsp.
- Large eggs - 3
- Almond milk - .25 cup
- Chopped nuts - ex. Hazelnuts – .25 cup
- Unsweetened almond/preference nut butter - .25 cup

How to Prepare:
1. Whisk all of the fixings in a container. Let the batter sit for 5-10 minutes so the flour will thicken.
2. Warm up a greased skillet (low-medium).
3. Measure out .25 cup portions of the batter in the frying pan. Cook for 2-3 minutes per side.

Meal Prep Tips:
1. Let the pancakes cool.

2. Pour the nuts into a baggie or plastic container. You can add the nuts in the containers together or separately.
3. You can store the pancakes for 5-7 days in the refrigerator.
4. Time to Eat: Warm up the pancakes and serve with the prepared almond butter drizzle.

Keto-Friendly Breakfast Beverages

These two options are a great incentive to get going with your meal prep, so just enjoy!

Bulletproof Coffee

Serving Yields: 1
Macros: 0 g Net Carbs | 320 Calories | 1 g Protein | 51 g Total Fats

Fixings Needed:
- MCT oil powder - 2 tbsp.
- Ghee/butter - 2 tbsp.

- Hot coffee - 1.5 cups

How to Prepare:
1. Empty the hot coffee into your blender.
2. Pour in the powder and butter. Blend until frothy.
3. Enjoy using a large mug.

Avocado Mint Green Smoothie

Serving Yields: 1
Macros: 5 g Net Carbs | 223 Calories | 1 g Protein |23 g Total Fats

Fixings Needed:
- Almond milk - .5 cup
- Full-fat coconut milk - .75 cup
- Avocado - .5 of 1 – approx. 3-4 oz.
- Cilantro - 3 sprigs
- Large mint leaves - 5-6
- Vanilla extract - .25 tsp.
- Lime juice - 1 squeeze
- Sweetener of your choice - to your liking
- Crushed ice - 1.5 cup

How to Prepare:

1. Measure each of the ingredients and add to your blender.
2. Combine on the low-speed setting until pureed.

Meal Prep Tips:

1. At this point, you can store in the fridge.
2. When you are ready to have the smoothie, just toss in the ice and mix.
3. Serve in a cold glass.

Blueberry Essence

Serving Yields: 1

Macros: 3 g Net Carbs | 343 Calories | 31 g Protein | 21 g Total Fats

Fixings Needed:

- Blueberries - .25 cup
- Coconut milk - 1 cup
- Whey protein powder (optional) - 1 scoop
- Vanilla Essence - 1 tsp.
- MCT Oil - 1 tsp.

How to Prepare:
1. For a quick burst of energy, add all of the fixings into a blender.
2. Puree until it reaches the desired consistency.

Meal Prep Tips:
1. Store in the fridge until ready to enjoy.
2. Add several chunks of ice if you like.

Blueberry Yogurt Smoothie

Serving Yields: 2
Macros: 2 g Net Carbs | 70 Calories | 2 g Protein | 5 g Total Fats

Fixings Needed:
- Blueberries - 10
- Yogurt - .5 cup
- Vanilla extract - .5 tsp.
- Coconut milk - 1 cup
- Stevia - to your liking

How to Prepare:
1. Add all of the fixings into the blender, mixing well.
2. When creamy, pour into 2 chilled mugs and enjoy.

Cinnamon Smoothie

Serving Yields: 1

Macros: 5 g Net Carbs | 467 Calories | 24 g Protein | 40.3 g Total Fats

Fixings Needed:
- Cinnamon - .5 tsp.
- Coconut milk - .5 cup
- Water - .5 cup
- Extra-virgin coconut oil/MCT oil - 1 tbsp.
- Ground chia seeds - 1 tbsp.
- Plain/vanilla whey protein - .25 cup
- Stevia drops - optional

How to Prepare:
1. Pour the milk, cinnamon, protein powder, and chia seeds in a blender.
2. Empty the coconut oil, ice, and water. Add a few drops of stevia to your liking.

Chapter 2

Tempting Lunchtime Choices

You have a wide variety to choose from, ranging from salads to soup and more.

Salad Choices

BLT Salad in a Jar

Serving Yields: 8
Macros: 7 g Net Carbs | 205 Calories | 17 g Protein |18 g Total Fats

Fixings Needed:
- Romaine Lettuce – 2 cups
- Iceberg Lettuce – 2 cups
- Chopped scallions – 2
- Diced tomatoes – 2
- Bacon slices – 4 crumbled

How to Prepare:
1. Combine all of the dressing ingredients.
2. Slowly pour into the jars.

3. Layer the veggies, croutons, and garnish of bacon.

Meal Prep Tips:
1. Tightly close each of the jars.
2. Store in the fridge for up to three days.

Caesar & Salmon Salad

Serving Yields: 2
Macros: 2 g Net Carbs | 466 Calories | 40 g Protein |32 g Total Fats

Fixings Needed:
- Salmon fillets – 2 – 6 oz. ea.
- Bacon – 4 slices
- Ghee – as needed – 1 tbsp.
- Freshly cracked black pepper – 1 pinch
- Pink salt – 1 pinch
- Sliced avocado – .5 of 1
- Romaine hearts – 2 cups chopped
- Caesar dressing – 2 tbsp.

How to Prepare:
1. Cook the bacon until crispy for 8 minutes using the med-high heat setting on the

stovetop. Drain on a platter using paper towels.

2. Remove the excess water from the fillets. Give them a shake of pepper and salt.
3. Use the same pan to prepare the salmon. Add butter if needed.
4. Cook for five minutes per side. This will be medium-rare.
5. Break the bacon into bits.

Meal Prep Tips:

1. Prepare two salad dishes or closed container for the meal prep with equal parts of romaine, avocado, and the bacon.
2. Place the bacon into separate containers to keep them crunchy.
3. When ready to serve, enjoy with a drizzle of the dressing.

Cauliflower & Citrus Salad

Serving Yields: 4
Macros: 1 Net Carbs | 177 Calories | 2 g Protein | 7 g Total Fats

Fixings Needed for the Salad:
- Small cauliflower – 1 - divided
- Small Romanesco cauliflower – 1 - divided
- Broccoli – 1 lb.
- Seedless oranges – 2

Fixings Needed for the Vinaigrette:
- Finely chopped anchovies – 4
- Orange – juice & zest – 1
- Salted – unrinsed capers – 1 tbsp.
- Finely chopped hot pepper – 1
- Pepper & Salt – to your liking
- Extra-virgin olive oil – 4 tbsp.

How to Prepare:
1. Cut the cauliflower into florets. Remove the peel and thinly slice the oranges. Finely chop the anchovies, capers, and hot peppers for the vinaigrette.
2. Prepare the vinaigrette fixings in a jar with a lid. Shake well and set aside.
3. Set up the Instant Pot with one cup of water and the steamer basket. Add the cauliflower to the basket and secure the lid. Set the timer for 6 minutes using low pressure. Quick-release the steam pressure when you hear the buzzer.

4. Transfer the florets to a serving dish with the prepared oranges. Toss.
5. Drizzle with the vinaigrette and enjoy.

Meal Prep Tips:
1. Prepare the salad and dressing.
2. Store in the fridge individually or in a large air-tight container.

Italian Tomato Salad

Serving Yields: 2
Macros: 6 g Net Carbs | 274 Calories | 14.1 g Protein | 22 g Total Fats

Fixings Needed:
- Minced garlic clove – 1
- Freshly chopped basil – .25 cup
- Olive oil – 2 tbsp.
- Balsamic vinegar – 1 tbsp.
- Pepper and salt – to taste
- Sliced ripe tomatoes – 2 Medium
- Fresh arugula – 3 cups
- Cubed mozzarella cheese – 3 oz.

How to Prepare:

1. Combine the oil, basil, garlic pepper, salt, and vinegar in a blender. Mix until smooth.
2. Toss the rest of the fixings in a salad container.

Meal Prep Tips:

Combine the salad and add the dressing mixture or add it to individual containers for an on-to-go method.

You can store this way for up to one day.

Kale Salad

Serving Yields: 4

Macros: 3 g Net Carbs | 80 Calories| 4 g Protein |6 g Total Fats

Fixings Needed:

- Kale – 1 bunch
- Lemon juice – 1 tbsp.
- Extra-virgin olive oil – 1 tbsp.
- Salt – .5 tsp.
- Parmesan cheese – .33 cup

How to Prepare:
1. Cut away the ribs from the kale and slice into ¼-inch strips. Store in a plastic bag or storage container until ready to eat.

Meal Prep Tips:
2. When you're ready to eat, just combine with the salt and oil, toss about 3 minutes until softened.
3. Combine the cheese, juice, and kale. Serve.

Rainbow Salad

Serving Yields: 8
Macros: 1 g Net Carbs |109 Calories | 15 g Protein | 9 g Total Fats

Fixings Needed for the Dressing:
- White balsamic vinegar – .5 cup
- Olive oil – 2 tbsp.
- Minced garlic cloves – 2
- Chopped parsley – .25 cup
- Salt & Pepper – 1 pinch

Fixings Needed for the Salad:

- Chopped red cabbage – 2 cups
- Assorted salad greens – 8 cups
- Chopped cucumber – 1 cup
- Sliced carrots – 1 cup
- Raw sunflower seeds – .5 cup
- Diced red bell pepper – 1
- Chopped yellow pepper – 1

How to Prepare:

1. Whisk all of the dressing fixings together. Pour into a serving container.
2. Drain the chickpeas and prep the veggies. Prepare the salads.

Meal Prep Tips:

1. You can refrigerate the salad for up to five days.
2. Pour the dressing into a closed jar and place in the fridge until it is dinner or lunch time.
3. Another Option: You can also add the dressing in the bottom of a mason jar with the salad fixings on top.

Time to Eat: Put the salad in individual dishes and pour on the dressing. If you used a jar, just shake and enjoy!

Thai Pork Salad

Serving Yields: 2
Macros: 5 g Net Carbs | 461 Calories | 29 g Protein | 33 g Total Fats

Fixings Needed for the Sauce:
- Juice & zest of 1 lime
- Chopped cilantro – 2 tbsp.
- Tomato paste – 2 tbsp.
- Soy sauce – 2 tbsp (+) 2 tsp.
- Red curry paste – 1 tsp.
- Five Spice – 1 tsp.
- Fish sauce – 1 tsp.
- Red pepper flakes – .25 tsp.
- Rice wine vinegar – 1 tbsp. (+) 1 tsp.
- Mango extract – .5 tsp.
- Liquid stevia – 10 drops

Fixings Needed for the Salad:
- Romaine lettuce – 2 cups
- Pulled pork – 10 oz.
- Medium chopped red bell pepper – .25 of 1
- Chopped cilantro – .25 cup

How to Prepare:
1. Zest half of the lime and chop the cilantro.
2. Mix all of the sauce fixings.

3. Blend the barbecue sauce components and set aside.
4. Pull the pork apart and make the salad. Pour a glaze over the pork with a bit of the sauce.

Meal Prep Tips:
1. Prepare the salad and sauce fixings.
2. Prepare the pork and shred.
3. Store in individual containers or in the fridge to use within a day or so.

Tuna Salad

Serving Yields: 2
Macros: 6 g Net Carbs | 465 Calories | 68.5 g Protein |18 g Total Fats

Fixings Needed:
- Fresh lemon juice – .5 of 1
- Olive oil – 1 tbsp.
- Large chopped boiled eggs – 2
- Tuna packed in oil – 2 cans – 15 oz.
- Sliced cucumber – .5 of 1
- Medium red onions – thinly sliced - 2
- Cilantro – .5 of 1

- Salt – 1 tsp.
- Dijon mustard – 2 tsp.
- Mayonnaise – 2 tbsp.

Meal Prep Tips:
1. Whisk the oil, lemon juice, mayo, and mustard in a container.
2. Drain the tuna and combine with the remainder the ingredients in another bowl.
3. Place each container in the fridge.
4. Ready to Eat: Add the dressing to the salad and toss to serve.

Soups

Chicken Pot Pie Soup

Serving Yields: 6
Macros: 3.5 g Net Carbs | 432 Calories | 20.5 g Protein |35 g Total Fats

Fixings Needed:
- Butter – 2 tbsp.
- Skinless – boneless chicken breasts – 1-1.5 lb.

- Small diced onion – .25 of 1
- Mixed veggies – .5 cup
- Chicken broth – 3 cups
- Black pepper – .25 tsp.
- Pink salt – .25 tsp.
- Minced cloves of garlic – 2
- Heavy whipping cream – 1.75 cups
- Cream cheese – 1 oz.
- Rosemary – .25 tsp
- Poultry seasoning – 1 tsp.
- Thyme – 1 pinch
- Xanthan gum – .5 tsp.

How to Prepare:
1. Melt the butter in the Instant Pot using the saute mode. Toss in the mixed veggies and onion. Cook a few minutes until translucent. Add them to a bowl and set to the side.
2. Deglaze the Instant Pot with 1/2 c. of the broth. Toss in the chicken along with the spices.
3. Close the top and select the poultry setting (15 min.). Natural release for six minutes and do a quick release of the rest of the pressure.

4. Shred the chicken and add the rest of the broth, chicken, cream cheese, veggies, and whipping cream into the pot.
5. Switch to the warm cycle and add the xanthan gum. Stir and saute about 10 minutes.

Meal Prep Tips:
1. Be sure to cool down the fixings completely.
2. Either store them in a covered glass dish or in individual dishes.
3. They will remain delicious for at least 2-3 days.

Zoodle Chicken Soup

Serving Yields: 2
Macros: 4 g Net Carbs | 310 Calories | 34 g Protein | 16 g Total Fats
Fixings Needed:
- Chicken broth – 3 cups
- Chicken breast – 1
- Avocado oil – 2 tbsp.
- Green onion – 1
- Celery stalk – 1

- Cilantro – .25 cup
- Salt – to taste
- Peeled zucchini – 1

How to Prepare:

1. Chop or dice the breast of the chicken. Pour the oil into a saucepan and cook the chicken until done. Pour in the broth and simmer. Chop the celery and green onions and toss into the pan. Simmer for 3-4 more minutes.
2. Chop the cilantro and prepare the zucchini noodles. Use a spiralizer or potato peeler to make the 'noodles.' Add to the pot.
3. Simmer for a few more minutes and season to your liking.

Meal Prep Tips:

1. Store in a glass container in the fridge. It will remain tasty for 2-3 days.

Pizza for Lunch

BBQ Meat-Lover's Pizza

Serving Yields: 2
Macros: 3.5 g Net Carbs | 18 g Protein | 27 g Total Fats

Fixings Needed:
- Mozzarella - 8 oz. – 2 cups
- Psyllium husk powder – 1 tbsp.
- Almond flour – .75 cup
- Cream cheese – 1.5 oz. - 3 tbsp.
- Large egg – 1
- Black pepper – .5 tsp
- Salt – .5 tsp.
- Italian seasoning – 1 tbsp.

Fixings Needed for the Topping:
- Mozzarella cheese – 4 oz. 1 cup
- BBQ sauce – to your liking
- Sliced Kabana/hard salami
- Bacon slices
- Sprinkled oregano – optional

How to Prepare:
2. Set the temperature of the oven to 400ºF.

3. Melt the cheese in the microwave – about 45 seconds. Toss in the cream cheese and egg, mixing well.
4. Blend in the psyllium husk, flour, salt, pepper, and Italian seasoning. Make the dough as circular as possible. Bake for ten minutes. Flip it onto a piece of parchment paper.
5. Cover the crust with the toppings. Sprinkle with more cheese.
6. Bake until the cheese is golden.

Meal Prep Tips:
1. According to your taste, you can cool the pizza thoroughly and slice.
2. Place in a freezer bag either as a whole or individually (if it makes it that far).

Beef & Pepperoni Pizza

Serving Yields: 4
Macros: 2 g Net Carbs | 610 Calories | 44 g Protein | 45 g Total Fats

Fixings Needed:
- Large eggs – 2

- Ground beef – 20 oz.
- Pepperoni slices – 28
- Pizza sauce – .5 cup
- Shredded cheddar cheese – .5 cup
- Mozzarella cheese – 4 oz.
- Also Needed: 1 Cast iron skillet

How to Prepare:
1. Combine the eggs, beef, and seasonings and place in the skillet to form the crust. Bake until the meat is done or about 15 minutes.
2. Take it out of the oven and add the sauce, cheese, and toppings. Place the pizza back in the oven a few more minutes until the cheese has melted.

Meal Prep Tips:
1. After it's cooled completely, slice the pizza into four equal portions for freezing.
2. You can also leave it whole and freeze. Add to a freezer bag until it's time to serve and enjoy.

Pita Pizza

Serving Yields: 2

Macros: 4 g Net Carbs | 250 Calories | 13 g Protein | 19 g Total Fats

Fixings Needed:
- Marinara sauce – .5 cup
- Low-carb pita – 1
- Cheddar cheese – 2 oz.
- Pepperoni – 14 slices
- Roasted red peppers – 1 oz.

How to Prepare:
1. Set the oven to 450ºF.
2. Slice the pita in half and put on a foil-lined baking tray. Rub with a bit of oil and toast for one to two minutes.
3. Pour the sauce over the bread, sprinkle with the cheese, and other toppings. Bake for another five minutes or until the cheese melts.

Meal Pep Tips:
1. Remove from the oven and let it cool thoroughly.
2. Store in the fridge for a couple of days.
3. Freeze to enjoy later using a freezer bag.

Seafood for Lunch

Cod Choices

Chili Lime Cod

Serving Yields: 2
Macros: 3 g Net Carbs | 215 Calories | 37 g
Protein | 5 g Total Fats

Fixings Needed:
- Wild-caught cod – 10-12 oz.
- Coconut flour – .33 cup
- Egg – 1
- Lime – 1
- Cayenne pepper – .5 tsp.
- Garlic powder – 1 tsp.
- Salt – 1 tsp.
- Crushed red pepper – 1 tsp.

How to Prepare:
1. Heat the oven temperature to reach 400ºF.
2. In separate dishes, whip the egg and remove any lumps from the flour.
3. Let the fillet soak in the egg dish for one minute on each side. Add it to the flour dish and then add it to a baking sheet.

4. Sprinkle the spices and drizzle the lime juice over the cod.
5. Bake 10 to 12 minutes or when it easily flakes apart.

Meal Pep Tips:
1. Cool completely once it is like you like it.
2. Wrap well in foil and store in the fridge for a day.
3. Freeze and enjoy later.
4. Once it is time to eat, just drizzle with some Sriracha if you wish, and enjoy.

Pan Fried Cod

Serving Yields: 4

Macros: 1 g Net Carbs | 160 Calories |21 g Protein |7 g Total Fats

Fixings Needed:
- Ghee – 3 tbsp.
- Cod fillets – 4
- Minced garlic cloves – 6
- Garlic powder – shake
- Salt – 1 pinch

How to Prepare:
1. Melt the ghee and add half of the garlic into a skillet.
2. Arrange the fillets in the pan using med-high heat. Sprinkle with the garlic pepper and the salt.
3. Once it turns white halfway up its side, turn it over and add the remainder of the minced garlic. Continue cooking until it flakes easily.

Meal Prep Tips:
1. Store a day or so or wrap up in foil and add to a plastic freezer bag for a longer time.
2. When ready to eat, serve with some ghee/garlic from the pan.

Salmon

Almond Pesto Salmon

Serving Yields: 2
Macros: 6 g Net Carbs | 610 Calories | 38 g Protein | 47 g Total Fats

Fixings Needed:
- Garlic clove - 1
- Almonds - .25 cup
- Olive oil - 1 tbsp.
- Lemon - .5 of 1
- Parsley - .5 tsp.
- Pink Himalayan salt - .5 tsp.
- Atlantic salmon fillets - 2 - 6 oz.
- Shallot - .5 of 1
- Lettuce - 2 handfuls
- Butter - 2 tbsp.

How to Prepare:
1. Make the Pesto: Pulse the almonds, garlic, and olive oil in the food processor to form a paste. Add the parsley, salt, and juice of the lemon. Set to the side.
2. Dry the salmon fillets and season them with a sprinkle of salt and pepper.
3. Cook the salmon four to six minutes (skin side down) in a lightly greased pan. Flip it and butter the pan to baste the fish for a minute or so (rare inside).

Meal Prep Tips:
1. Store the pesto in the fridge.
2. When the salmon is done, cool entirely. Store in the fridge overnight or freeze for later.

3. When ready to eat, just serve over some lettuce with a dollop of pesto, slivered almonds, and shallots.

Creamy Salmon & Pasta

Serving Yields: 2
Macros: 3 g Net Carbs | 470 Calories | 21 g Protein |42 g Total Fats

Fixings Needed:
- Coconut oil – 2 tbsp.
- Zucchinis - 2
- Smoked salmon – 8 oz.
- Mayo – keto-friendly - .25 cup

How to Prepare:
1. Use a peeler or spiralizer to make noodle-like strands from the zucchini.
2. Warm up the oil over the med-high temperature setting. When hot, add the salmon and saute 2-3 minutes until golden brown.
3. Stir in the noodles and saute 1-2 more minutes.

Meal Prep Tips:

1. Store the noodles in the fridge after cooled overnight.
2. When it's time to eat, just stir in the mayo and divide the pasta between two dishes.
3. Serve and enjoy!

Chapter 3

<u>Dinner Favorites</u>

Beef Choices

Balsamic Beef Pot Roast

Serving Yields: 10
Macros: 3 g Net Carbs |393 Calories|30 g
Protein |28 g Total Fats

Fixings Needed:
- Ground black pepper – 1 tsp.
- Kosher salt – 1 tbsp.
- Garlic powder – 1 tsp.
- Boneless chuck roast – 3 lb.
- Balsamic vinegar - .25 cup
- Chopped onion - .5 cup
- Water – 2 cups
- Xanthan gum - .25 tsp.
- For the Garnish: Chopped fresh parsley

How to Prepare:
1. Slice the roast in half and season with the garlic powder, pepper, and salt.

53

2. Prepare the pot using the saute function and brown the meat.
3. Pour in the onion, water, and vinegar. Secure the lid and set for 35 minutes. Natural release the pressure in the Instant Pot.
4. Add the meat to a container and break it apart. Discard fat and use the saute function to simmer the juices in the pot. Add the beef back after whisking in the xanthan gum. Gently stir and turn off the heat.

Meal Prep Tips:
1. Let the roast cool completely.
2. Store it in a heavy-duty freezer bag.
3. Thaw and warm it up. Garnish as desired.

Cumin Spiced Beef Wraps

Serving Yields: 2
Macros: 4 g Net Carbs | 375 Calories | 30 g Protein | 26 g Total Fats

Fixings Needed:
- Coconut oil – 1-2 tbsp.
- Diced onion – .25 of 1
- Ground beef - .66 lb.
- Chopped cilantro – 2 tbsp.
- Red bell pepper – 1 diced
- Minced ginger – 1 tsp.
- Cumin – 2 tsp.
- Minced garlic cloves – 4
- Pepper and salt - to taste
- Large cabbage leaves - 8

How to Prepare:
1. Warm up a frying pan and pour in the oil.
2. Saute the peppers, onions, and ground beef using medium heat.
3. When done, add the pepper, salt, cumin, ginger, cilantro, and garlic.

Meal Prep Tips:
1. Cool the burger entirely and add to storage containers.

Time to Eat:
2. Prepare the Leaves: Fill a large pot with water (3/4 full) and wait for it to boil. Cook each leaf for 20 seconds, plunge it

in cold water and drain before placing it on your serving dish.
3. Reheat the beef mixture.
4. Scoop the mixture onto each leaf, fold, and enjoy.

Sweet and Sour Meatballs

Serving Yields: 5
Macros: 5 g Net Carbs | 295 Calories | 28 g Protein | 18.7 g Total Fats

Fixings Needed:
- Large egg - 1
- Ground beef – 1 lb.
- Onion powder - .5 tsp.
- Parmesan cheese - .25 cup

Fixings Needed for the Sauce:
- Soy sauce – 3 tbsp.
- Water – 1.5 cups
- Apple cider vinegar - .25 cup
- Erythritol – 1 cup
- Sugar-free ketchup - .33 cup
- Xanthan gum - .5 tsp.

How to Prepare:
1. Use your hands to combine the egg, beef, onion powder, and parmesan cheese in a mixing container. Shape the mixture into about thirty balls.
2. Add the meatballs to a heated saucepan and brown. Set them aside.
3. Pour in the soy sauce, water, vinegar, Erythritol, and ketchup using the same pan and stir.
4. Slowly, pour in the xanthan gum, but be sure to wait a couple of minutes in between pouring to be sure it thickens. Lower the temperature to low and simmer. Check the sauce every two minutes until it reaches the desired texture.

Meal Prep Tips:
1. You can add the sauce into the meatballs if you will be using the recipe within a day or so.
2. Or just simmer the sauce. Store the sauce and meatballs individually. Portion into 5 individual containers.
3. When ready to eat, just add the meatballs and sauce into a pan. Simmer for ten minutes on low.

Tasty Short Ribs

Serving Yields: 4

Macros: 2.5 g Net Carbs | 685 Calories | 25.7 g Protein |62 g Total Fats

Fixings Needed:
- Keto-friendly soy sauce - .25 cup
- Beef short ribs – 6 – 4 oz. each
- Rice vinegar – 2 tbsp.
- Fish sauce – 2 tbsp.
- Red pepper flakes - .5 tsp.
- Sesame seeds - .5 tsp.
- Onion powder - .5 tsp.
- Minced garlic - .5 tsp.
- Ground ginger – 1 tsp.
- Salt – 1 tbsp.
- Cardamom - .25 tsp.

How to Prepare:
1. Mix the fish sauce, vinegar, and alternative soy sauce.
2. Arrange the ribs in a dish with high sides. Add the sauce and marinate for up to 1 hour.
3. Combine all of the spices together. Take the ribs from the dish and sprinkle with the rub.
4. Warm up the grill (med-high) and cook for 3 to 5 minutes on each side.

Meal Prep Tips:
1. Put the ribs in a platter to cool.
2. Place in freezer bags or into plastic containers (4 portions) until it's time to serve and enjoy.

Chicken Choices

Authentic Butter Chicken

Serving Yields: 6
Macros: 6 g Net Carbs | 293 Calories | 25 g Protein | 17 g Total Fats

Fixings Needed:
- Chicken breast – 1.5 lb.
- Garam masala – 2 tbsp.
- Grated fresh ginger – 3 tsp.
- Minced garlic – 3 tsp.
- Plain yogurt – 4 oz.
- Coconut oil - 1 tbsp.

Fixings Needed for the Sauce:
- Ghee or butter – 2 tbsp.
- Onion - 1
- Fresh ginger - grated – 2 tsp.

- Minced garlic – 2 tsp.
- Crushed tomatoes - 14.5 oz.
- Ground coriander – 1 tbsp.
- Garam masala - .5 tbsp.
- Chilli powder – 1 tsp.
- Cumin – 2 tsp.
- Heavy cream - .5 cup
- Salt – to your liking

Optional Toppings:
- Cilantro
- Cauliflower rice

How to Prepare:
1. In a large dish, use a sharp knife and dice the chicken breasts into 2-inch pieces. Stir in 2 tablespoons garam masala, 1 teaspoon grated ginger, and 1 teaspoon minced garlic. Add in the yogurt, stir to combine. Chill at least 30 minutes.
2. For the Sauce: Place the onion, ginger, garlic, crushed tomatoes, and spices in a blender. Pulse until creamy smooth. Place the sauce to the side for now.
3. Warm up the oil in a good-sized pan using the medium-high heat setting. Arrange the chicken in the skillet,

browning 3 to 4 minutes per side. Once browned, pour in the sauce, cook 5 to 6 minutes longer.
4. Stir in the heavy cream and ghee, continue to cook another minute. Taste for salt and add additional if needed. Top with cilantro and serve with cauliflower rice if desired.
5. Note: Nutritional information does not include cauliflower rice.

Meal Prep Tips:
1. Prepare the chicken and place into the storage container of choice. Store in the fridge or freezer – with the container clearly marked.
2. Prepare the sauce and place in baggies unless you are planning on using quickly. If you are serving within several days, just prepare and store it in an airtight container.
3. When ready to prepare, just continue with step 4, combining the cream and ghee with the chicken, etc.

Buffalo Chicken Burgers

Serving Yields: 2 burgers
Macros: 1 g Net Carbs | 488 Calories | 43 g Protein | 34 g Total Fats

Fixings Needed:
- Chicken breasts – 8 oz. cooked
- Room-temperature cream cheese - 2 oz.
- Shredded mozzarella cheese - .5 cup
- Frank's Red-Hot Sauce or your choice – 2 tbsp.
- Coconut oil or ghee for frying

How to Prepare:
1. Either chop or shred the prepared chicken and combine with the rest of the fixings.
2. Place the fixings in the microwave for 15 to 20 seconds to help compact the ingredients. Form two medium patties and place on a plate. Store in the freezer for about 15 minutes.
3. Warm up a skillet using the high heat setting. Add the fat and patties. Prepare the burgers for 2 to 3 minutes per side.
4. Serve when crispy brown.

Meal Prep Tips:
1. Prepare the chicken and mix to form patties.
2. Freeze or cook and freeze the patties.

Chicken and Asparagus Pan Dinner

Serving Yields: 8
Macros: 4 g Net Carbs | 439 Calories | 63 g Protein | 18.2 g Total Fats

Fixings Needed:
- Chicken breasts – 4 lbs.
- Avocado oil – 1 tbsp.
- Trimmed asparagus – 1 lb.
- Sun-dried tomatoes - 4
- Thick-cut bacon – 4 slices
- Salt – 1 tsp.
- Pepper - .25 tsp.
- Provolone cheese – 8 slices
- Also Needed: 1 baking pan

How to Prepare:
1. Slice the chicken into 8 thin pieces. Chop the bacon and tomatoes into one-inch pieces.

2. Warm up the oven temperature to 400ºF.
3. Add the oil to the baking pan along with the chicken and asparagus. Top it off with the tomatoes and bacon. Sprinkle some pepper and salt for seasoning.
4. Bake until the chicken reaches 160ºF internally or about 25 minutes.
5. Toss in the asparagus and cheese.
6. Garnish with some bacon and tomatoes. Bake another three to four minutes until the cheese has melted.

Meal Prep Tips:
1. Simply prepare the chicken and store in the fridge for several days.
2. Place into plastic bins or freezer bags until ready to use.
3. Prepare the asparagus when ready to eat and combine with the cheese. Garnish and serve.

Chicken & Bacon Patties

Serving Yields: 10 Patties
Macros: 1.5 g Net Carbs | 95.6 Calories | 7.25 g Protein | 6.16 g Total Fats

Fixings Needed:

- Bacon – 4 slices
- Chicken breast – 1 can – 12 oz.
- Medium bell peppers - 2
- Large egg - 1
- Sun-dried tomato pesto - .25 cup
- Parmesan cheese - .25 cup
- Coconut flour – 3 tbsp.

How to Prepare:

1. In the food processor, finely chop the peppers and add them to a mixing container. Use a paper towel to pat the excess liquid from the veggies after mixing.
2. Prepare the bacon – cook until crispy. Cool and chop it with the chicken. Add it to the processor until almost smooth. Combine all of the fixings and make patties.
3. Fry on the med-hi to the medium setting in a skillet with a little oil.
4. Once browned on one side, flip it and continue cooking until done. Let the grease drain on the towels.

Meal Prep Tips:

1. Let them cool completely. Store in the fridge for a day or so.

2. Store in freezer bags and place in the freezer for later. Be sure to mark its contents clearly.
3. When it is time to eat, just garnish with your favorite toppings but remember to count the extras.

Chicken & Gravy

Serving Yields: 2
Macros: 4 g Net Carbs | 375 Calories | 30 g Protein | 26 g Total Fats

Fixings Needed:
- Coconut oil – 1-2 tbsp.
- Diced onion – .25 of 1
- Ground beef - .66 lb.
- Chopped cilantro – 2 tbsp.
- Red bell pepper – 1 diced
- Minced ginger – 1 tsp.
- Cumin – 2 tsp.
- Minced garlic cloves – 4
- Pepper and salt - to taste
- Large cabbage leaves - 8

How to Prepare:

1. Warm up a frying pan and pour in the oil.
2. Saute the peppers, onions, and ground beef using medium heat.
3. When done, add the pepper, salt, cumin, ginger, cilantro, and garlic.

Meal Prep Tips:

1. Cool the burger entirely and add to storage containers.

Time to Eat:

2. Prepare the Leaves: Fill a large pot with water (3/4 full) and wait for it to boil. Cook each leaf for 20 seconds, plunge it in cold water and drain before placing it on your serving dish.
3. Reheat the beef mixture.
4. Scoop the mixture onto each leaf, fold, and enjoy.

Chicken Kiev

Serving Yields: 2
Macros: 4 g Net Carbs | 510 Calories|50 g Protein |33 g Total Fats

Fixings Needed:
- Breasts of chicken – 2 – 6 oz. each
- Cloves of garlic - 2
- Butter – 4 tbsp.
- Green onion – 1 stalk
- Parsley - pinch
- Tarragon - pinch
- Pepper and salt – to taste
- Pork rinds – 1 oz.
- Coconut flour - .25 cup
- Egg - 1

How to Prepare:
1. Set the oven temperature to 350ºF.
2. Use a tenderizing hammer to pound the chicken until they are approximately one-half-inch to one-inch thick. Flavor it with the tarragon, pepper, salt, and parsley.
3. Add chopped bits of butter, garlic, and green onion evenly to the pieces of chicken. Close with toothpicks.
4. Crush the pork rinds for the crumbs (NutriBullet for a few seconds works great.)
5. Make dredging dishes, one each for flour, a beaten egg, and the pork rind crumbs.
6. Cover the chicken with the flour, egg, then the rinds. Close them tightly with a

toothpick. Let the fixings chill in the fridge for about ½ hour.
7. Fry the breasts until browned on all sides in a lightly oiled pan.
8. Transfer and arrange them in a baking dish.
9. Bake for approximately 20 minutes. Baste with any leftover butter.

Meal Prep Tips:
1. Let the chicken cool completely. Store in the fridge for one to two days.
2. You can also portion the fixings into freezer bags and store for later.
3. When ready to serve, add to a bed of lettuce.

Chicken Parmesan

Serving Yields: 2
Macros: 3 g Net Carbs | 600 Calories | 74 g Protein | 32 g Total Fats

Fixings Needed:
- Breasts of chicken – 1 lb.
- Parmesan cheese – 2 tbsp.

- Pork rinds – 1 oz.
- Egg – 1
- Marinara sauce - .5 cup
- Shredded mozzarella - .5 cup

Possible Garnish Ingredients:
- Garlic powder
- Oregano
- Freshly cracked black pepper
- Salt

How to Prepare:
1. Program the oven temperature to 350ºF.
2. Use a food processor/Magic Bullet to crush the pork rinds and parmesan cheese. Add them to a bowl.
3. Pound the chicken breasts until they are ½-inch thick. Beat the egg and dip the chicken in for an egg wash. Dip the chicken into the crumbs.
4. Arrange the breasts on a baking sheet that is lightly greased. Sprinkle with the seasonings and bake for 25 minutes.

Meal Prep Tips:
1. When done, just cool the prepared chicken. Store in the fridge for a day or

so. After that time, add to a freezer bag or storage container awaiting a side dish.
2. Time to Serve: Pour the marinara sauce over each portion. Garnish with the mozzarella and bake for 15 minutes.
3. Enjoy with spinach.

Pork Choices

Asian-Inspired Pork Chops

Serving Yields: 4
Macros: 3 g Net Carbs | 327.4 Calories| 41.3 g Protein | 15.6 g Total Fats

Fixings Needed:
- Pork chops – boneless -4
- Cloves of garlic – 4 halved
- Lemongrass – peeled and diced – 1 stalk
- Star anise – 1 medium
- Almond flour – 1 tbsp.
- Fish sauce – 1 tbsp.
- Sambal chili paste - .5 tbsp.
- Sugar-free ketchup - .5 tbsp.
- Soy sauce – 1.5 tsp.

- Sesame oil – 1 tsp.
- Peppercorns - .5 tsp.
- Five Spice - .5 tsp.

How to Prepare:

1. Pound the chops until they are about ½ - inch thick.
2. Slice the garlic into halves. Grind the star anise and peppercorns with a pestle and mortar or in a blender. Toss in the garlic and lemongrass. Mix until pureed and add the soy sauce, five spice powder, sesame oil, and fish sauce. Stir well.
3. Place the chops in a baking pan, add the marinade, and coat well. Cover for one to two hours at room temperature.
4. Lightly coat the chops with the flour and add to a pan set on the high-heat setting. Sear about two minutes on each side. Place on the cutting board and chop into several strips.
5. Make a sauce by combining the ketchup and chili paste. Yummy!

Meal Prep Tips:

1. Prepare the chops and place into containers or freezer bags or store in the fridge or freezer – your choice.
2. Prepare the sauce on the day you are ready to serve or store it in 4 individual containers for added convenience.

Chicken Fried Pork Chops

Serving Yields: 4
Macros: 0.8 g Net Carbs |390 Calories| 28.8 g Protein |20.8 g Total Fats

Fixings Needed:
- Bone-out pork chops – 4 medium - 16 oz. ea.
- Ground pork rinds – 1 oz.
- Chopped nuts – 1 tbsp.
- Flaxseed meal – 2 tbsp.
- Salt – 1 tsp.
- Almond flour – 2 tbsp.
- Large egg - 1
- Oil or fat of choice – 4 tbsp.

How to Prepare:

1. In a food processor, grind the rinds to a powder and combine with the flaxseed meal, flour, and nut blend.
2. Warm up the oil/fat in a skillet using the med-hi setting.
3. Whisk an egg in a dish and dip the chop. Dip in the rind mixture (step 1). Coat well and fry for about four to five minutes for each side. The internal temperature should reach 145ºF.
4. Serve and enjoy!

Meal Prep Tips:
1. This one is easy for meal prep. All you need to do is prepare the chops and store in the freezer bag or in the fridge for tomorrow — your choice.

Pan-Fried Pork Chops

Serving Yields: 3
Macros: 4 g Net Carbs | 385 Calories | 22.1 g Protein | 27 g Total Fats

Fixings Needed:

- Coconut flour - .5 cup
- Salt and black pepper – 1 tsp. each
- Pork chops - 3
- Butter – 1 tbsp.

How to Prepare:

Combine all of the dry fixings in a large mixing container.

Pat the chops dry with a paper towel.

Melt the butter in a skillet on the stovetop.

Cover the chops with the mixture and prepare each side for 4 to 5 minutes.

Serve with your favorite side dishes.

Meal Prep Tips:

1. Once the chops have finished cooking. Let them cool completely.
2. Place them in an air-tight container and use within a couple of days.
3. You can also place them individually in freezer bags for later. Be sure to date and mark the preparation method.

Parmesan Crusted Pork Chops

Serving Yields: 14

Macros: 3 g Net Carbs | 354 Calories | 33 g Protein | 34 g Total Fats

Fixings Needed:
- Parmesan cheese – 6 oz.
- Pork chops - 14
- Large eggs - 2
- Almond flour - .75 cup
- Pepper and salt – to your liking
- For Frying: Bacon grease

How to Prepare:
1. Heat up the oven to 400ºF.
2. Grate the parmesan and mix with the flour and spices.
3. Whisk the eggs in a shallow dish.
4. Dip the chops in the eggs, then the parmesan mixture.
5. Fry in the bacon grease on each side for one minute.
6. Arrange on a baking dish in the oven, bake until done.

Meal Prep Tips:

1. Store safely in the fridge for several days.
2. Place in freezer bags and store. Make sure you date and add the name of the recipe to recall it later.

Pulled Pork

Serving Yields: 8
Macros: 2.2 g Net Carbs |464 Calories| 43 g Protein | 30.2 g Total Fats

Fixings Needed:
- Boneless pork shoulder – 3 lb.
- Chopped white onion - 1
- Bay leaves - 3
- Smoked paprika – 1 tsp.
- Pink Himalayan salt – 3 tsp.
- Garlic powder – 2 tsp.

How to Prepare:
1. Heat up the slow cooker using the low setting. Combine the paprika, salt, and garlic powder. Slice the pork into chunks and rub into the spices.
2. Chop the onion and toss it into the cooker along with the pork. Add the bay

leaves and close the lid. Cook for 10
hours on low.
3. When ready, shred and let cool.

Meal Prep Tips:
1. Add the shredded pork to individual bags
   for the freezer or into compartmentalized
   dishes to await a veggie.
2. Be sure to date the containers and label
   with the name of its content.

Chapter 4

Sides - Snacks & Appetizers

For most of the side veggie dishes, it is usually best to prepare no more than 24 hours ahead of time (unless otherwise noted in the recipe). You can use these delicious sides any time.

Sides

Asparagus & Garlic

Serving Yields: 4
Macros: 2 g Net Carbs | 61 Calories | 1 g Protein | 6 g Total Fats

Fixings Needed:
- Minced garlic – 1 tbsp.
- Fresh asparagus – 1 bunch
- Butter – 2 tbsp.

How to Prepare:
1. Rinse the asparagus and separate each of the stalks. Boil them for 2-3 minutes. Drain and chill in a dish of cold water.

2. Warm up the garlic and butter in a skillet. Fry the asparagus with them until browned.

Meal Prep Tips:
1. Once they are cooled, you can store them in one dish.
2. You can also divide them into individual containers with other choices for later.

Baked Radishes & Brown Butter Sauce

Serving Yields: 2
Macros: 2 g Net Carbs | 181 Calories | 1 g Protein | 19 g Total Fats

Fixings Needed:
- Olive oil – 1 tbsp.
- Halved radishes – 2 cups
- Butter – 2 tbsp.
- Freshly ground black pepper & Pink Himalayan salt – to taste
- Freshly chopped flat-leaf Italian parsley – 1 tbsp.

How to Prepare:
1. arm up the oven to reach 450ºF.
2. Cut the radishes into halves and toss into the oil. Sprinkle with the pepper and salt. Spread them on a baking sheet – single layered. Bake for 15 minutes. Stir about halfway through the cycle.
3. After they have roasted 10 minutes, use the medium heat setting on the stovetop to melt the butter mixed with the salt. Simmer until it's a nutty brown (3 min.). Pour the butter into a mug and set aside.

Meal Prep Tips:
1. Let everything cool completely. Take the radishes out of the oven and portion into two plates.
2. You can divide the butter into two containers or leave in one container for a day or two.
3. When ready to serve. Heat up and add the butter and top it off with the fresh parsley.

Buffalo Cauliflower Bites

Serving Yields: 4

Macros: 3 g Net Carbs | 130 Calories | 2 g Protein | 12 g Total Fats

Fixings Needed:
- Cauliflower florets – 4 cups
- Cracked black pepper – to taste
- Sea salt - .25 tsp.
- Cayenne pepper - .25 tsp.
- Salted butter – 4 tbsp.
- Hot sauce - .25 cup
- Minced garlic – 1 clove
- Paprika - .25 tsp
- Optional – Blue cheese dressing

How to Prepare:
1. Warm up the oven until it reaches 375ºF.
2. Arrange the florets on a paper-lined baking tray.
3. Whisk the cayenne, black pepper, salt, paprika, garlic, butter, and hot sauce. Pour into a microwavable-safe dish for 30 seconds or until smooth.
4. Empty the sauce over the florets in the pan and bake for 25 minutes.

Meal Prep Tips:
1. Cool thoroughly. Add to individual containers or freezer bags.
2. You can store in the fridge for a couple of days.
3. Serve with a bowl of blue cheese dressing for dipping.

Caprese Salad

Serving Yields: 4

Macros: 5 g Net Carbs | 191 Calories | 7.7 g Protein | 63.5 g Total Fats

Fixings Needed:
- Grape tomatoes – 3 cups
- Peeled garlic cloves - 4
- Avocado oil – 2 tbsp.
- Mozzarella balls – 19 pearl-sized
- Baby spinach leaves – 4 cups
- Fresh basil leaves - .25 cup
- Brine reserved from the cheese – 1 tbsp.
- Pesto - 1 tbsp.

How to Prepare:
1. Use a sheet of aluminum foil to cover a baking tray.
2. Set the oven temperature setting to 400ºF.
3. Arrange the cloves and tomatoes on the baking pan and drizzle with the oil. Bake for 20-30 minutes until the tops are slightly browned.
4. Drain the liquid (saving one tablespoon) from the mozzarella. Mix the pesto with the brine.
5. Arrange the spinach in a large serving bowl. Transfer the tomatoes to the dish along with the roasted garlic.

Meal Prep Tips:
- Cool the ingredients thoroughly. Place in closed containers until time to use.
- Drizzle with the pesto sauce. Garnish with the mozzarella balls and freshly torn basil leaves.

Cauliflower Mac & Cheese

Serving Yields: 4

Macros: 7 g Net Carbs | 294 Calories | 11 g Protein | 23 g Total Fats

Fixings Needed:

- Butter – 3 tbsp.
- Cauliflower – 1 head
- Cheddar cheese – 1 cup
- Black pepper & sea salt - to taste
- Unsweetened almond milk - .25 cup
- Heavy cream - .25 cup

How to Prepare:

1. Slice the cauliflower into small florets and shred the cheese.
2. Heat up the oven to reach 450ºF. Use a piece of aluminum foil or parchment paper to line a baking sheet.
3. Melt 2 tbsp. of butter. Toss the florets and butter. Give it a shake of pepper and salt. Place the cauliflower on the baking pan and roast 10-15 minutes.
4. Warm up the rest of the butter, milk, heavy cream, and cheese in the microwave or double boiler.
5. Pour on the cheese.

Meal Prep Tips:
1. Prepare the mac and cheese and let it cool thoroughly.
2. Store in an airtight container to use within a day or so.
3. Warm up and serve.

Cobb Salad

Serving Yields: 2
Macros: 3 g Net Carbs | 600 Calories| 43 g Protein | 48 g Total Fats

Fixings Needed:
- Hard-boiled egg - 1
- Spinach – 1 cup
- Bacon strips - 2
- Campari tomato - .5 of 1
- Chicken breast – 2 oz.
- Avocado - .25 of 1
- Olive oil – 1 tbsp.
- White vinegar - .5 tsp.

How to Prepare:
1. Prepare the bacon and chicken shred or slice the chicken.

2. Cut all of the ingredients into small pieces. Toss them to a bowl.

Meal Prep Tips:
1. You can add the prepared salad into individual bowls and securely close with a lid.
2. When it is time to eat, drizzle with the vinegar and oil.
3. Toss gently and serve.

Hibachi Mushrooms – Japanese Style

Serving Yields: 4
Macros: 3 g Net Carbs |102 Calories| 3.4 g Protein | 8.9 g Total Fats

Fixings Needed:
- Unsalted butter – 3 tbsp.
- White onion, diced - .5 of 1
- Button mushrooms, halved or quartered – 8 oz.
- Tamari – 3 tbsp.
- Pepper – 0.125 tsp.
- Salt – to your liking

How to Prepare:
1. Heat the butter over medium-high heat in a 10.5" cast iron skillet.
2. Stir in onion and mushrooms. Saute for about 5 minutes then add in tamari, continue to cook until the sauce has almost evaporated.

Meal Prep Tips:
1. Season with salt to taste. Let them cool completely.
2. You can portion them into a freezer baggie or plastic container for freezer storage. Be sure to remove the air from the chosen container.
3. You can also place them in the fridge in a closed container to use within a day or so.

Lemony Green Beans with Almonds

Serving Yields: 4

Macros: 6.5 g Net Carbs |131 Calories| 3.5 g Protein | 9.8 g Total Fats

Fixings Needed:
- Lemon juice – 1-2 tbsp.
- Unrefined sea salt - .5 tsp
- Garlic cloves - 4
- Fresh green beans – 1 lb.
- Sliced organic almonds - .33 cup
- Olive oil– 2 tbsp.

How to Prepare:
1. Trim the beans and steam until tender and crispy. Add the salt and lemon juice - toss gently.
2. Warm up the olive oil in a pan using the med-low setting. Blend in the almonds and cook until the almonds start changing colors and add the garlic. Continue cooking for 30 seconds. Cook the garlic no more than 60 seconds because it will lose its nutrients.
3. Mix everything together and toss well.

Meal Prep Tips:
1. Prepare the recipe. Let it cool completely.
2. If you have a container system for your prep, add it to another dish.
3. You can also store it in an individual container for the freezer or in a regular dish for serving in the next day or so.

Snack Choices

Healthy Chia Bars

Serving Yields: 14

Macros: 1.5 g Net Carbs | 121 Calories| 2.5 g Protein | 11 g Total Fats

Fixings Needed:
- Toasted almonds - .5 cup
- Coconut oil – divided – 1 tbsp. (+) 1 tsp.
- Erythritol – 4 tbsp. - divided
- Butter - 2 tbsp.
- Heavy cream - .25 tsp.
- Liquid stevia - .25 tsp.
- Vanilla extract – 1.5 tsp.
- Unsweetened & shredded coconut flakes - .5 cup
- Chia seeds - .25 cup
- Coconut cream - .5 cup
- Coconut flour – 2 tbsp.
- Also Needed: Food Processor

How to Prepare:
1. Add the toasted almonds into the food processor and pulse until crumbly.
2. Toss in 1 tablespoon of the coconut oil and 2 tablespoons of the erythritol.

Continue processing until you have almond butter. (Now you have another new usable product.)

3. Warm up a pan and add the butter, heavy cream, erythritol, stevia, and vanilla. Stir until they're bubbly and fold in the almond butter. Stir to blend.

4. In a blender, grind the chia seeds to make a powdery mix. In another pan, toast the coconut flakes and mix with the chia seeds. Melt the coconut cream in a separate skillet.

5. Now, combine all of the fixings and add the melted coconut cream, flour, and coconut oil. Store in the fridge for one hour.

Meal Prep Tips:
1. When it's ready, slice into squares and store in the refrigerator.
2. For convenience, you can place them into individual dishes or freezer bags.

Peanut Butter Protein Bars

Serving Yields: 12 Bars

Macros: 3 g Net Carbs |172 Calories| 7 g Protein | 14 g Total Fats

Fixings Needed:
- Keto-friendly chunky peanut butter – 1 cup
- Egg whites - 2
- Almonds - .5 cup
- Cashews - .5 cup
- Almond meal – 1.5 cups

How to Prepare:
1. Warm up the oven ahead of time to 350ºF.
2. Combine all of the fixings and add to the prepared dish.
3. Bake for 15 minutes and cut into 12 pieces once they're cooled.

Meal Prep Tips:
1. Store in the fridge to keep them fresh.

Fat Bombs

Almond Butter Fat Bombs

Serving Yields: 8
Macros: 1.7 g Net Carbs | 145 Calories|1.5 g Protein | 14.7 g Total Fats

Fixings Needed:
- Almond butter – 9.5 tbsp.
- Melted coconut oil - .75 cup
- Liquid stevia – .25 tsp. or to your taste
- Melted salted butter – 9 tbsp.
- Cocoa – 3 tbsp.

How to Prepare:
2. Combine all of the components listed until smooth.
3. Add the final product to 24 mini muffin molds or use silicone candy molds.

Meal Prep Tips:
1. Freeze for a minimum of 30 minutes or until frozen solid for prep.
2. Pop them out and enjoy. Store in the freezer in an airtight container or zipper freezer baggie.

Blueberry Cream Cheese Fat Bombs

Serving Yields: 12

Macros: 1 g Net Carbs |67 Calories| 0.96 g Protein | 7.4 g Total Fats

Fixings Needed:
- Cream cheese – 1.5 cups
- Fresh or frozen berries – 1 cup
- Swerve – 2-3 tbsp.
- Vanilla extract – 1 tbsp.
- Coconut oil - .5 cup

How to Prepare:
1. For 30 to 60 minutes before preparation time, place the cream cheese on the countertop to become room temperature.
2. Take the stems off the berries and rinse. Pour into a blender. Mix well until smooth.
3. Pour in the Swerve and extract. Blend in the oil and cream cheese.
4. Add the mixture to candy molds and freeze for approximately two hours.

Meal Prep Tips:

1. Once the bombs are solid, just pop them out.
2. Store in freezer bags or another safe freezer container.

Chocolate Fat Bombs

Serving Yields: 24
Macros: 1 g Net Carbs | 180 Calories|3 g Protein | 21 g Total Fats

Fixings Needed:
- Coconut oil - .5 cup
- Splenda or your preference – 3 packets
- Walnut or almond butter - .25 cup
- Sugar-free coffee liqueur syrup – ex. Da Vinci – 2 tbsp.
- Heavy whipping cream - .25 cup
- Walnut halves - 24
- Also Needed: Silicon molds

How to Prepare:

1. Use a glass measuring cup and add the oil, walnut butter, coffee liqueur, cocoa powder, and sweetener.
2. Microwave for 30-40 seconds. Stir the contents until the oil melts.
3. Stir in the cream and pour into the molds. Arrange a nut in each one.

Meal Prep Tips:
1. Freeze the bombs until solid.
2. Leave them in the molds or pop them out and add them to a storage or container.
3. If you are planning a trip, add a bunch to individual serving bags for a quick snack.

Coffee Fat Bombs

Serving Yields: 15
Macros: -0- g Net Carbs | 45 Calories| -0- g Protein | 4 g Total Fats

Fixings Needed:
- Cream cheese – room temperature – 4.4 oz.
- Powdered Xylitol – 2 tbsp.
- Instant coffee – 1 tbsp.

- Coconut oil – 1 tbsp.
- Unsweetened cocoa powder – 1 tbsp.
- Room temperature butter – 1 tbsp.

How to Prepare:
1. Take the butter and cream cheese out of the fridge about an hour before it's time to begin.
2. With a blender/food processor, blitz the xylitol and coffee into a fine powder. Add the hot water to form a pasty mix.
3. Blend in the butter, cream cheese, cocoa powder, and coconut oil.
4. Add to ice cube trays and freeze a minimum of one to two hours.

Meal Prep Tips:
1. Use Ziplock bags to keep them fresh in the freezer.

Lemonade Fat Bombs

Serving Yields: 2
Macros: 7 g Net Carbs | 404 Calories| 4 g Protein | 43 g Total Fats

Fixings Needed:

- Cream cheese – 4 oz.
- Butter – 2 oz.
- Lemon zest & juice - .5 of 1 lemon
- Swerve - 2 tsp.
- Pink Himalayan salt – 1 pinch or to taste

How to Prepare:
2. Take the butter and cream cheese out of the fridge and let it become room temperature before using. Zest the lemon and juice it into a small dish.
3. In another container, mix the butter with the cream cheese. Use a hand mixer to combine all of the fixings until well mixed.
4. Spoon the mixture into small molds or cupcake paper liners in a muffin tin pan.
5. Stick the chosen holder in the freezer for two hours.

Meal Prep Tips:
1. Take them out of the molds and put them in a zipper-top baggie to enjoy any time.
2. Store in the freezer for up to three months.

<u>Appetizers</u>

Chicken Salad Deviled Eggs

Serving Yields: 6
Macros: 2 g Net Carbs | 128 Calories| 13 g Protein | 7 g Total Fats

Fixings Needed:
- Old Bay Seasoning – 1 dash
- Lemon pepper – .5 tsp.
- Dill - .5 tsp.
- Celery salt – 1 pinch
- Chopped onion – 1 tbsp.
- Dijon mustard – 1 tsp.
- Mayonnaise – 2 tbsp.
- Shredded chicken – 1 cup
- Large eggs – 6

How to Prepare:
1. Combine all of the fixings, omit the eggs, and store in the fridge for later.
2. Gently place the eggs in a pot of water (just enough to cover the eggs).
3. Set the temperature on high until it boils and lower the setting to medium.
4. Boil for 15 minutes and transfer to cool under cold running water.

5. Remove the shell and slice the eggs into halves. Remove the yolk and fill with the salad mixture. Sprinkle with the old bay seasoning.
6. Note: Discard the yolks or use in another recipe. Total time is just 30 minutes.

Meal Prep Tips:
1. These eggs are a great solution for those times when you want to entertain your guests or just want a goodie to add to your dinner tray.
2. Just make a batch and see how quickly they disappear.

Little Smokies

Serving Yields: 12
Macros: 3.3 g Net Carbs |177 Calories| 7.3 g Protein | 15.1 g Total Fats

Fixings Needed:
- Cocktail Smokies – 24 oz.
- Avocado oil – 2 tbsp.
- Fixings Needed for the BBQ Sauce:
- Unsweetened ketchup – 1 cup
- Water - .5 cup

- Apple cider vinegar – 3 tbsp.
- Brown swerve - .25 cup
- Worcestershire sauce – 1 tsp.
- Natural maple flavoring – 2 tsp.
- Dijon mustard – 1 tsp.
- Salt - .5 tsp.
- Garlic powder - .5 tsp
- Black pepper - .25 tsp.
- Onion powder - .5 tsp
- Also Needed: 1 iron skillet

How to Prepare:

1. Combine the sauce fixings in a jar or other container and set to the side for now.
2. Warm up the oil in the skillet using the med-high heat setting.
3. Sear the smokies for 2 to 3 minutes until they begin to change color.
4. Stir in the sauce and lower the heat to simmer for (10 to 15 min.) or until thickened to your liking.
5. Note: The average serving size is 6, but it will depend on the brand used. (Trader Joe's Cocktail Pups were used in this one.)

Meal Prep Tips:
1. This is a great choice to prep for a party. Just prepare a day or so before the party and you are ready to go!
2. Freeze if you want to save them for later. They should be good for up to one to two months. If they're constantly frozen at 0ºF, they should last indefinitely.

Condiments – The Keto-Friendly Way

Condiments are the items that can cause issues with your new way of eating using keto techniques. Problems may arise of how to remain in ketosis and still enjoy the dining condiments that are offered in most supermarkets. The short answer is – you cannot. Are you wondering how to prepare that keto-friendly meal? The answer is simple. This segment is a special bonus for some of those times when nothing else will work in your favorite keto recipe. These are so delicious that you will not realize they are very healthy choices. Keep your ketosis in line with one of these favorites:

Keto-Friendly Dips & Sauces

For the easiest prep for your dips and sauces, just prepare each choice and store according to the recipe.

Lemon-Dill Tartar Sauce

Serving Yields: 1
Macros: 1 g Net Carbs |85 Calories| -0- g Protein | 9 g Total Fats

Fixings Needed:
- Mayonnaise – 1 cup
- Dill pickles – 2
- Dill pickle juice - 1 tbsp.
- Freshly squeezed lemon juice - .5 tsp.
- Sea salt – 1 pinch
- Onion powder - .5 tsp.
- Black pepper- to taste

How to Prepare:
1. Combine all of the fixings.

2. You can store the sauce in an air-tight container for up to three days.

Ketchup

Macros: 1.1 g Net Carbs |9 Calories| -0- g Protein | -0- g Total Fats

Fixings Needed:
- Diced tomatoes – 1 can organic – 14.5 oz. (+) 1 can water
- Italian seasoning – 1 tsp.
- Star anise – 1 piece
- White vinegar - .5 tbsp.
- Freshly ground pepper
- Salt
- Optional: Erythritol – to your liking

How to Prepare:
1. In a small saucepan, add the tomatoes and add a can of water.
2. Stir in the herbs and anise. Simmer using the low heat setting for one hour, stirring frequently.

3. Transfer the pan from the heat and add the vinegar. Add any other seasonings as desired and remove the star anise.
4. Let it cool and puree into a smooth ketchup sauce using a blender/food processor.

Meal Prep Tips:
1. Store in the fridge for no more than 4 days.

<u>Mayonnaise</u>

Avocado Mayo

Serving Yields: 4

Macros: 4 g Net Carbs | 1 g Protein | 5 g Total Fats
Fixings Needed:
- Avocado - .5 of 1 medium
- Pink salt – 1 pinch
- Ground cayenne pepper - .5 tsp.
- Lime juice - .5 of 1
- Olive oil - .25 cup

How to Prepare:

2. Dice the avocado and toss into a blender or food processor. Pulse and add in the salt, cayenne, cilantro, and lime juice.
3. When smooth, stir in the oil – 1 tbsp. at a time -
4. You can store the mayo for up to one week in a sealed glass bottle.

Sriracha Mayo

Serving Yields: 4

Macros: 2 g Net Carbs|1 g Protein | 22 g Total Fats

Fixings Needed:

- Sriracha sauce – 2 tbsp.
- Paprika - .25 tsp.
- Mayonnaise - .5 cup
- Onion - .5 tsp.
- Garlic - .5 tsp.

How to Prepare:

1. Whisk the fixings together in a small container.
2. It will store easily for up to one week in the fridge.

Salad Dressings

Blue Cheese Chunky Style Dressing

Serving Yields: 4
Macros: 3 g Net Carbs | 7 g Protein | 32 g Total Fats

Fixings Needed:
- Mayonnaise - .5 cup
- Sour cream - .5 cup
- Lemon juice - .5 of 1
- Worcestershire sauce - .5 tsp.
- Black pepper and salt – to your liking
- Crumbled blue cheese – 2 oz.

How to Prepare:
1. Whisk all of the fixings except for the cheese until well mixed.
2. Fold in the cheese gently and store in a closed glass dish for up to one week.

Caesar Dressing

Serving Yields: 4
Macros: 2 g Net Carbs |2 g Protein | 23 g Total Fats

Fixings Needed:
- Mayonnaise - .5 cup
- Dijon mustard – 1 tbsp.
- Lemon juice - .5 of 1
- Worcestershire sauce - .5 tsp.
- Parmesan cheese - .25 cup
- Freshly cracked black pepper – 1 pinch
- Pink Himalayan salt – to taste

How to Prepare:
1. Whisk the lemon juice, mustard, mayonnaise, salt, pepper, and Worcestershire sauce. Stir well and add the parmesan.
2. Whisk until smooth.
3. You can store up to one week in a glass container in the fridge.

Chapter 5

<u>Desserts</u>

Find yourself a tasty ketogenic treat in this segment that is fit for a king or queen!

<u>**Brownie Muffins**</u>

Serving Yields: 6
Macros: 4.4 g Net Carbs | 183 Calories| 7 g Protein |13 g Total Fats

Fixings Needed:
- Salt - .5 tsp.
- Flaxseed meal – 1 cup
- Cocoa powder - .25 cup
- Cinnamon – 1 tbsp.
- Baking powder - .5 tbsp.
- Coconut oil – 2 tbsp.
- Large egg - 1
- Vanilla extract – 1 tsp.
- Sugar-free caramel syrup - .25 cup
- Pumpkin puree - .5 cup
- Slivered almonds - .5 cup

- Apple cider vinegar – 1 tsp.

How to Prepare:
1. Set the oven temperature to 350ºF.
2. Use a deep mixing container — mix all of the fixings and stir well.
3. Use 6 paper liners in the muffin tin and add 1/4 cup of batter to each one.
4. Sprinkle several almonds on the tops, pressing gently.
5. Bake approximately 15 minutes or when the top is set.

Meal Prep Tips:
1. Cut the brownies into six portions.
2. Store in plastic baggies for the fridge or freezer bags if you want to have them last longer than 3-4 days.

<u>Cheesecake Cupcakes</u>

Serving Yields: 12
Macros: 2.1 g Net Carbs | 204 Calories| 5 g Protein | 20 g Total Fats

Fixings Needed:
- Almond meal – .5 cup
- Melted butter – .25 cup
- Eggs – 2
- Softened cream cheese – 2 – 8 oz. pkg.
- Stevia or your favorite sweetener – .75 cup
- Vanilla extract – 1 tsp.

How to Prepare:
1. Warm up the oven until it reaches 350ºF. Prepare a muffin tin with 12 paper liners.
2. Combine the butter and almond meal. Spoon into the cups to make a flat crust.
3. Whisk the vanilla, sweetener of choice, eggs, and cream cheese with an electric mixer until creamy. Scoop it in on top of the crust.
4. Bake for 15-17 minutes.

Meal Prep Tips:
1. Once they're done the cooking cycle, just remove and cool at room temperature.
2. You can store them overnight or at least 8 hours in the fridge.
3. Enjoy anytime for a delicious treat.

Cinnamon Apples – Instant Pot

Serving Yields: 4 large dishes
Macros: 2 g Net Carbs |110 Calories| 9 g Protein | 3 g Total Fats
Fixings Needed:
- Brown sugar - .5 cup - keto-friendly substitute
- Sugar - .5 cup or Swerve – 2 tsp.
- Cinnamon – 1 tbsp.
- Nutmeg - .125 tsp.
- Unsalted butter – 2 tbsp.
- Cornstarch – 3 tbsp.
- Granny Smith apples – 6
- Salt – 1 pinch

How to Prepare:
1. Peel and slice the apples thin.
2. Combine all of the fixings in the Instant Pot. Press the manual function for 18 minutes. Natural release the pressure (10 min.) and open the pot.
3. Stir and serve or prep.
4. Note: The macro totals are calculated using regular sugar and brown sugar.

Meal Prep Tips:
1. Let the apples cool to room temperature. Store in an airtight container or heavy-duty freezer bags.
2. Refrigerate for up to 7 days.
3. You can keep the apples fresh in the freezer for about 2 months.

Delicious No-Bake Coconut Cookies

Serving Yields: 20

Macros: -0- g Net Carbs | 99 Calories| 3 g Protein |10 g Total Fats

Fixings Needed:
- Melted coconut oil – 1 cup
- Monk fruit sweetened maple syrup or sweetener of choice - .5 cup
- Shredded unsweetened coconut flakes – 3 cups

How to Prepare:
1. Cut out a sheet of parchment paper and place on a cookie tray.

2. Combine all of the fixings. Run your hands through some water from the tap and shape the mixture into small balls. Arrange them on the pan around one to two inches apart.
3. Press them down to form a cookie and refrigerate until firm.

Meal Prep Tips:
1. You can prepare these into individual bags if you're an on-the-go kind of person.
2. The cookies will remain fresh covered for up to 7 days at room temperature.
3. Store in the fridge for up to a month.
4. If you choose, you can freeze the cookies for up to two months.

Mocha Cheesecake Bars

Serving Yields: 16
Macros: 3 g Net Carbs | 232 Calories| 6 g Protein | 21 g Total Fats

Fixings Needed for the Brownie Layer
- Vanilla extract – 2 tsp.
- Unsalted butter – 6 tbsp.
- Large eggs - 3
- Almond flour – 1.5 cups
- Hershey's Baking Cocoa - .5 cup
- Erythritol – 1 cup
- Salt - .5 tsp.
- Instant coffee - .5 tbsp.
- Baking powder – 1 tsp.

Fixings Needed for the Cream Cheese Layer
- Erythritol - .5 cup
- Softened cream cheese – 1 lb.
- Large egg - 1
- Vanilla extract – 1 tsp
- Also Needed: 8x8-inch baking pan

How to Prepare:
1. Warm up the oven to 350ºF. Lightly grease or spray the pan with a spritz or oil cooking spray.
2. Combine the wet fixings starting with the vanilla and butter and mix in the eggs.
3. In another container, combine the dry ingredients and whisk with the wet

fixings. Set aside 1/4 cup of the batter for later. Pour the mixture into the pan.

4. Mix the cream cheese (room temperature) with the rest of the ingredients for the second layer. Spread it on the layer of brownies.

5. Use the reserved batter as the last layer (will be thin). Bake 30-35 minutes.

Meal Prep Tips:

1. When cooled, slice the cheesecake bars.

2. Store in the fridge for several days or freeze in containers or freezer bags for extended use. Be sure to date and add the name of the contents.

Peanut Butter Fudge

Serving Yields: 18

Macros: -0- g Net Carbs |89 Calories| 2 g Protein | 8 g Total Fats

Fixings Needed:

- Peanut butter - .5 cup
- Coconut oil - .5 cup

- Sweetener of choice – ex. liquid stevia granulated sweetener – to taste
- Also Needed: 12-18 count muffin tin & liners or a loaf pan

How to Prepare:
1. Prepare the tin of choice with some cooking spray or a spritz of oil.
2. Combine the oil and peanut butter together on the stovetop or microwave. Melt and add the sweetener.

Meal Prep Tips:
1. Scoop the mixture into the tins or loaf pan and freeze.
2. You can serve with some (optional) melted chocolate – but count the carbs. Enjoy your treat anytime.

Spice Cakes

Serving Yields: 12
Macros: 3 g Net Carbs | 277 Calories| 6 g Protein | 27 g Total Fats

Fixings Needed:
- Eggs - 4
- Baking powder – 2 tsp.
- Almond flour – 2 cups
- Salted butter - .5 cup
- Nutmeg - .5 tsp.
- Allspice - .5 tsp.
- Ginger - .5 tsp.
- Cinnamon - .5 tsp
- Erythritol - .75 cup
- Ground cloves - .25 tsp.
- Vanilla extract – 1 tsp.
- Water – 5 tbsp.

How to Prepare:
1. Set the temperature in the oven to 350ºF. Prepare a cupcake tray with liners (12).
2. Mix the butter and erythritol with a hand mixer. Once it's smooth, combine with 2 eggs and the vanilla. Mix and stir in the remainder of the eggs, stirring until creamy.
3. Grind the clove to a fine powder and add with the rest of the spices. Whisk into the mixture. Stir in the baking powder and almond flour. Blend in the water. When

the batter is smooth, add to the prepared tin.
4. Bake for 15 minutes. Enjoy any time.

Meal Prep Tips:
1. Cool thoroughly for the prep.
2. Store in the fridge for a few days or in the freezer to enjoy later.
3. Be sure to label it with the date and its contents accurately.

Vanilla Cinnamon Protein Bites

Serving Yields: 18-20 bites
Macros: 4 g Net Carbs |112 Calories| 2 g Protein | 9 g Total Fats

Fixings Needed:
- Nut butter of choice - .25 - .33 cup
- Pure maple syrup - .25 - .33 cup
- Protein powder – vanilla - .25 cup
- Almond meal - .5 cup
- Vanilla extract - .5 – 1 tsp.
- Quick oats - .75 cup
- Cinnamon – 1 tbsp.

- Also Needed: Food processor

How to Prepare:

1. Line a cookie tin with a layer of parchment paper.
2. Grind the oats with the processor and add to a mixing container. Combine the cinnamon, protein powder, almond meal, and nut butter.
3. Mix in the syrup and vanilla. Using your hands, mix well and roll into small balls.
4. Freeze for 20-30 minutes.
5. Arrange in a Ziplock-type baggie with the cinnamon and vanilla protein.

Meal Prep Tips:

1. After dusting the bites, store in the fridge for three weeks.
2. Store in the freezer for up to six months.

Conclusion

Hopefully, you have found many new ways to prepare meals for you and your family. I would like to provide you with a few ideas to carry with you as you proceed using meal prep and your ketogenic techniques for dieting.

- Think long-term of how keto will work for you.
- Keep your intake of carbs low.
- Prepare a food journal and familiarize yourself with an online app to remain in ketosis with ease.
- Gather a food list of your favorite spices and other products to convert your pantry to keto.
- Begin using your new diet plan, remembering you can adjust the menu plan using the carbohydrate limitations you have each day.

You have all of the tools to be successful, but you still need to understand how to test to ensure you are in ketosis. Your individual progress can be tested using several items to ensure you remain in a ketogenic state. They include testing your breath, blood, or urine.

Take a blood test. It is recommended by the American Diabetes Association to test your blood using the blood ketone meter, particularly during times you are ill. Add a small drop of blood on a testing strip and insert the tab into the meter. It will indicate the amount of beta-hydroxybutyrate in your bloodstream. The results are highly accurate and consistent. Unfortunately, the strips are expensive and if you are squeamish of needles, this is not for you.

Test your breath. A Ketonix meter will provide you with a way to test your breath for ketosis. You just breathe into the meter to receive a special coded color. You will compare those colors with a guideline strip provided in the package. It is less messy, but it does take longer to get a reading.

Test your urine. One huge advantage of testing our urine is that the strips are inexpensive and can detect acetoacetate - one of the ketone bodies. The strip is dipped into the urine which will change the color of the strip. The various shades of purple and pink will clearly indicate the levels of the ketones. The darker the color on the testing strip, the higher the level of ketones. Early morning testing provides the most accurate score after a ketogenic diet dinner the evening before testing.

However, long-term testing with the strips is not as accurate as other methods. It can be misleading since the acetoacetate will only show up if they are in excessive levels. As your body adapts to ketosis, it will use the acetoacetate and the levels would read lower even if you're in ketosis.

There is no time like the present to gather your lists of goods needed to begin your ketogenic way of living. Begin with your food and prep items and before you know it, you will be prepping your freezer to the maximum with all the delicious keto foods your body is craving.

If you have a few moments, I would appreciate a review on Amazon if you found your new book useful in any way. Enjoy your new way of living!

*If You have a few moments, I would appreciate a review on **Amazon**, if You found your new book useful in any way.*

Enjoy!

© Copyright 2021 by **TAMARA GREEN**

<u>All Rights Reserved</u>

CPSIA information can be obtained
at www.ICGtesting.com
Printed in the USA
BVHW041013150321
602551BV00006B/454